KETO PESCATARIAN COOKBOOK FOR WEIGHT LOSS

Lose Weight Almost Effortlessly With The Best Seafood Recipes

KetonUSA

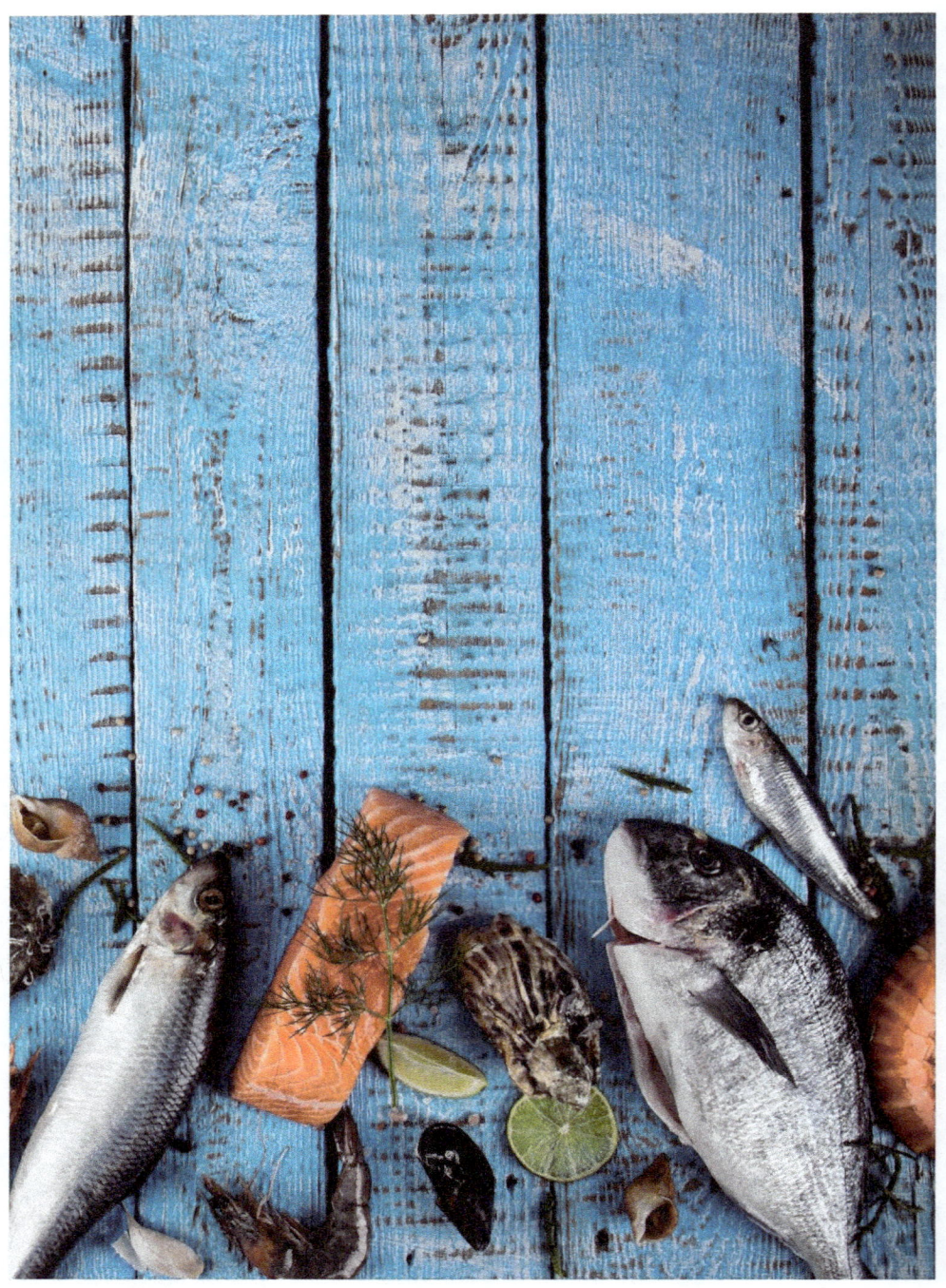

© Copyright 2021 by KetonUSA- All rights reserved. The following Book is reproduced below with the goal of providing information that is as accurate and reliable as possible. Regardless, purchasing this Book can be seen as consent to the fact that both the publisher and the author of this book are in no way experts on the topics discussed within and that any recommendations or suggestions that are made herein are for entertainment purposes only. Professionals should be consulted as needed prior to undertaking any of the action endorsed herein. This declaration is deemed fair and valid by both the American Bar Association and the Committee of Publishers Association and is legally binding throughout the United States. Furthermore, the transmission, duplication, or reproduction of any of the following work including specific information will be considered an illegal act irrespective of if it is done electronically or in print. This extends to creating a secondary or tertiary copy of the work or a recorded copy and is only allowed with the express written consent from the Publisher. All additional right reserved. The information in the following pages is broadly considered a truthful and accurate account of facts and as such, any inattention, use, or misuse of the information in question by the reader will render any resulting actions solely under their purview. There are no scenarios in which the publisher or the original author of this work can be in any fashion deemed liable for any hardship or damages that may befall them after undertaking information described herein.Additionally, the information in the following pages is intended only for informational purposes and should thus be thought of as universal. As befitting its nature, it is presented without assurance regarding its prolonged validity or interim quality. Trademarks that are mentioned are done without written consent and can in no way be considered an endorsement from the trademark holder.

Table of Contents

THE HEALTHY .... ERRORE. IL SEGNALIBRO NON È DEFINITO.

LOSE WEIGHT ALMOST EFFORTLESSLY WITH THE BEST SEAFOOD RECIPES 1

- FISH AND SEAFOOD MAIN DISHES 8
- TASTY AIR FRIED COD 9
- DELICIOUS CATFISH 12
- GRAPES SALAD 14
- TABASCO SHRIMP 16
- LEMONY SABA FISH 18
- ASIAN HALIBUT 19
- COD AND VINAIGRETTE 21
- SHRIMP AND CRAB MIX 23
- SEAFOOD CASSEROLE 25
- TROUT FILLET AND ORANGE SAUCE 28
- COD FILLETS AND PEAS 30
- THYME AND PARSLEY SALMON 32
- TROUT AND BUTTER SAUCE 34
- CREAMY SALMON 36
- SALMON & AVOCADO SALSA 38
- ITALIAN BARRAMUNDI FILLETS AND TOMATO SALSA 41
- CREAMY SHRIMP AND VEGGIES 43
- STUFFED CALAMARI 46
- SALMON AND CHIVES VINAIGRETTE 48
- HALIBUT AND SUN DRIED TOMATOES MIX 50
- BLACK COD AND PLUM SAUCE 52
- FISH AND COUSCOUS 55
- CHINESE COD 57
- COD WITH PEARL ONIONS 59
- HAWAIIAN SALMON 60
- SALMON AND AVOCADO SALAD 62
- SALMON AND GREEK YOGURT SAUCE 65
- SPECIAL SALMON 67
- SPANISH SALMON 69
- MARINATED SALMON 71
- DELICIOUS RED SNAPPER 73
- SNAPPER FILLETS AND VEGGIES 75
- AIR FRIED BRANZINO 77
- LEMON SOLE AND SWISS CHARD 79
- SALMON AND BLACKBERRY GLAZE 81
- ORIENTAL FISH 83

DELICIOUS FRENCH COD	85
SPECIAL CATFISH FILLETS	87
COCONUT TILAPIA	89
TILAPIA AND CHIVES SAUCE	91
HONEY SEA BASS	93
TASTY POLLOCK	95
BUTTERED SHRIMP SKEWERS	98
ASIAN SALMON	100
COD STEAKS WITH PLUM SAUCE	102
FLAVORED AIR FRIED SALMON	104
SALMON WITH CAPERS AND MASH	106

Fish & Seafood Main Dishes

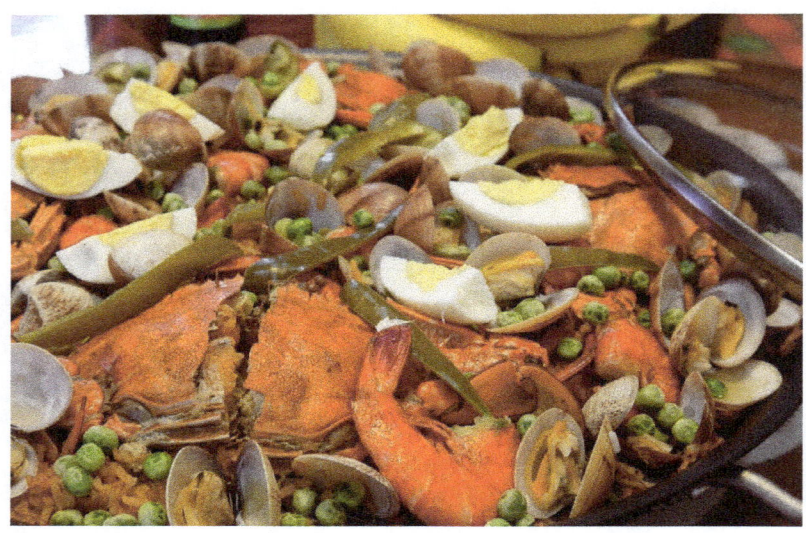

Get ready to dive into a sea of delicious recipes! Fish is one of the best sources of omega-3 fatty acids, which can help fight inflammation and heart disease, and it's a great source of protein to help keep your muscles strong while you're on a ketogenic diet. Still, despite the flavor and health benefits, seafood is not the easiest cuisine to prepare. Enter the air fryer. The air fryer will be your favorite tool for creating fresh and delicious, perfectly crisp fish and seafood recipes. From Fried Tuna Salad Bites to Firecracker Shrimp, you'll soon be a master of seafood cuisine, creating flavorful dishes your amily can't get enough of!

Tasty Air Fried Cod

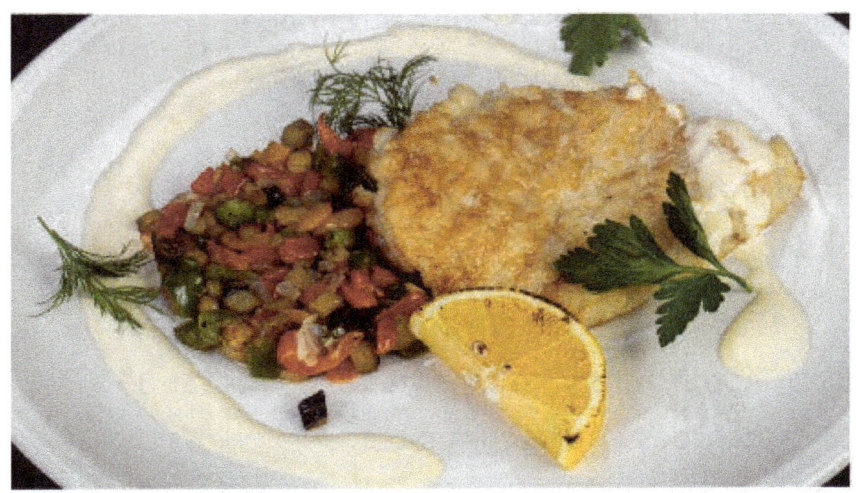

Preparation time: 10 minutes

Cooking time: 12 minutes

Servings: 4

Ingredients:

- 2 cod fish, 7 ounces each
- A drizzle of sesame oil
- Salt and black pepper to the taste 1 cup water
- 1 teaspoon dark soy sauce
- 4 tablespoons light soy sauce
- 1 tablespoon sugar

- 3 tablespoons olive oil
- 4 ginger slices
- 3 spring onions, chopped
- 2 tablespoons coriander, chopped

Directions:

√ Season fish with salt, pepper, drizzle sesame oil, rub well and leave aside for 10 minutes.
√ Add fish to your air fryer and cook at 356 degrees F for 12 minutes.
√ Meanwhile, heat up a pot with the water over medium heat, add dark and light soy sauce and sugar, stir, bring to a simmer and take off heat.
√ Heat up a pan with the olive oil over medium heat, add ginger and green onions, stir, cook for a few minutes and take off heat.
Divide fish on plates, top with ginger and green onions, drizzle soy sauce mix, sprinkle coriander and serve right away.

Enjoy!

Nutrition: calories 300, fat 17, fiber 8, carbs 20, protein 22

Delicious Catfish

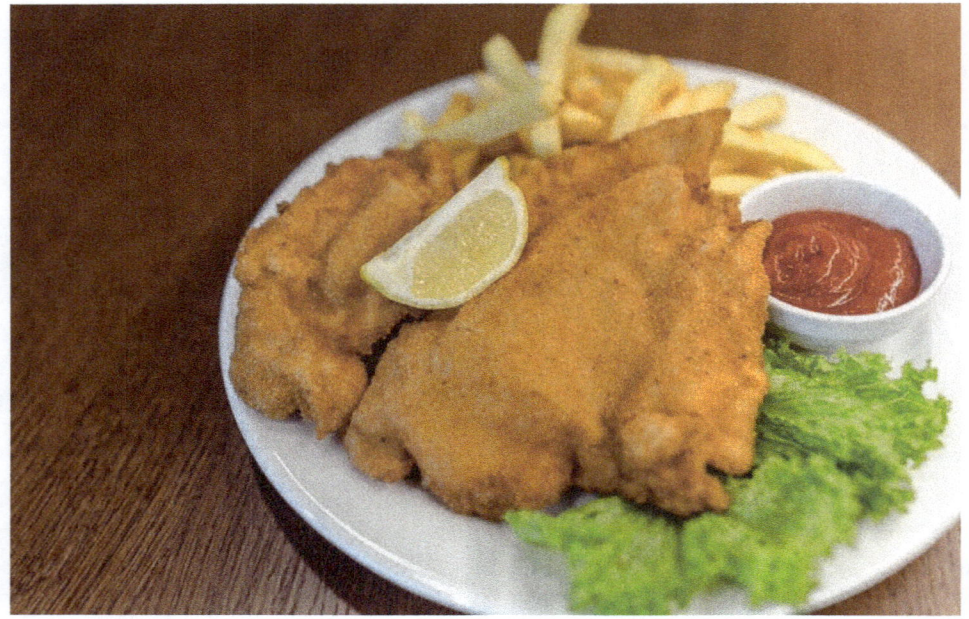

Preparation time: 10 minutes

Cooking time: 20 minutes

Servings: 4

Ingredients:

- 4 cat fish fillets
- Salt and black pepper to the taste A pinch of sweet paprika

- 1 tablespoon parsley, chopped
- 1 tablespoon lemon juice
- 1 tablespoon olive oil

Directions:

√ Season catfish fillets with salt, pepper, paprika, drizzle oil, rub well, place in your air fryer's basket and cook at 400 degrees F for 20 minutes, flipping the fish after 10 minutes.

√ Divide fish on plates, drizzle lemon juice all over, sprinkle parsley and serve. Enjoy!

Nutrition: calories 253, fat 6, fiber 12, carbs 26, protein 22

Grapes Salad

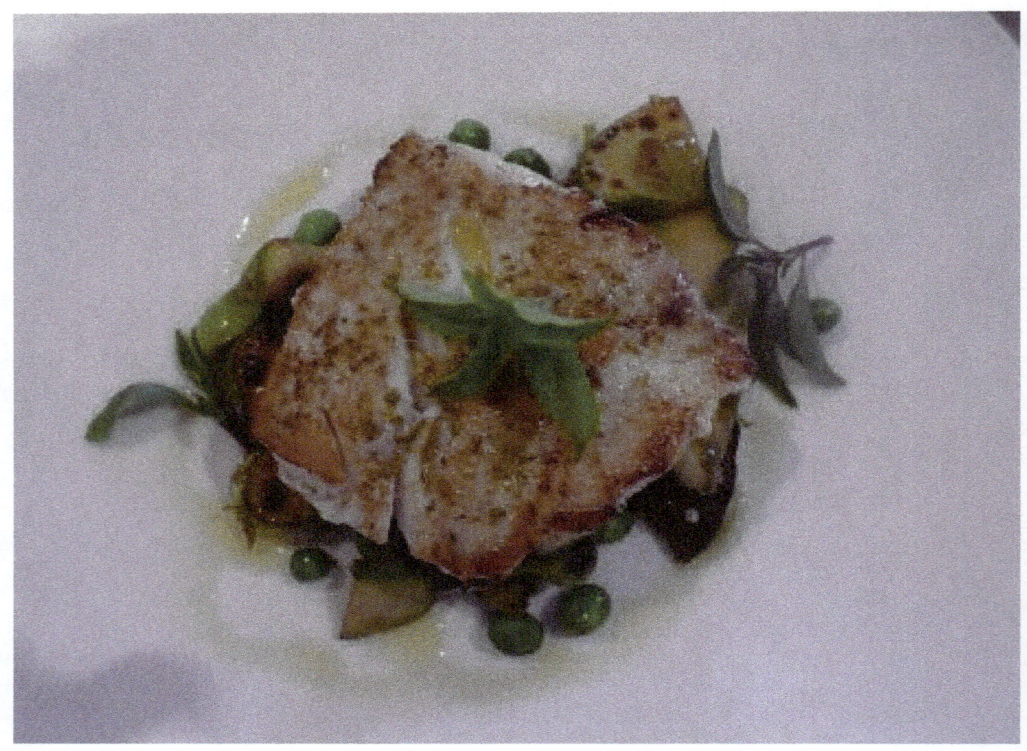

Preparation time: 10 minutes

Cooking time: 15 minutes

Servings: 2

Ingredients:

- 2 black cod fillets, boneless

- 1 tablespoon olive oil
- Salt and black pepper to the taste 1 fennel bulb,
- thinly sliced
- 1 cup grapes, halved
- 1/2 cup pecans

Directions:

√ Drizzle half of the oil over fish fillets, season with salt and pepper, rub well, place fillets in your air fryer's basket, cook for 10 minutes at 400 degrees F and transfer to a plate.

√ In a bowl, mix pecans with grapes, fennel, the rest of the oil, salt and pepper, toss to coat, add to a pan that fits your air fryer and cook at 400 degrees F for 5 minutes.

√ Divide cod on plates, add fennel and grapes mix on the side and serve.

Enjoy!

Nutrition: calories 300, fat 4, fiber 2, carbs 32, protein 22

Tabasco Shrimp

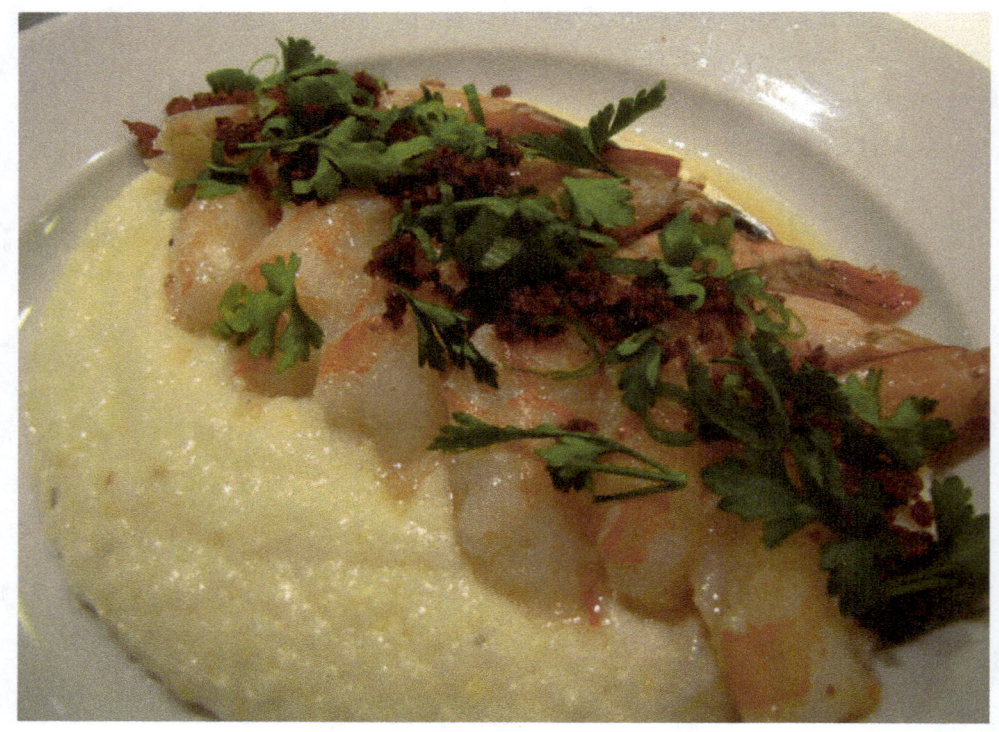

Preparation time: 10 minutes

Cooking time: 10 minutes

Servings: 4

Ingredients:

- 1 pound shrimp, peeled and deveined 1 teaspoon red pepper flakes

- 2 tablespoon olive oil
- 1 teaspoon Tabasco sauce
- 2 tablespoons water
- 1 teaspoon oregano, dried
- Salt and black pepper to the taste 1/2 teaspoon parsley, dried
- 1/2 teaspoon smoked paprika

Directions:

√ In a bowl, mix oil with water, Tabasco sauce, pepper flakes, oregano, parsley, salt, pepper, paprika and shrimp and toss well to coat.

√ Transfer shrimp to your preheated air fryer at 370 degrees F and cook for 10 minutes shaking the fryer once.

√ Divide shrimp on plates and serve with a side salad. Enjoy!

Nutrition: calories 200, fat 5, fiber 6, carbs 13, protein 8

Lemony Saba Fish

Preparation time: 10 minutes

Cooking time: 8 minutes

Servings: 1

Ingredients:

- 4 Saba fish fillet, boneless
- Salt and black pepper to the taste 3 red chili pepper, chopped
- 2 tablespoons lemon juice
- 2 tablespoon olive oil
- 2 tablespoon garlic, minced

Directions:

√ Season fish fillets with salt and pepper and put in a bowl.
√ Add lemon juice, oil, chili and garlic toss to coat, transfer fish to your air fryer and cook at 360 degrees F for 8 minutes, flipping halfway.
√ Divide among plates and serve with some fries.

Enjoy!

Nutrition: calories 300, fat 4, fiber 8, carbs 15, protein 15

Asian Halibut

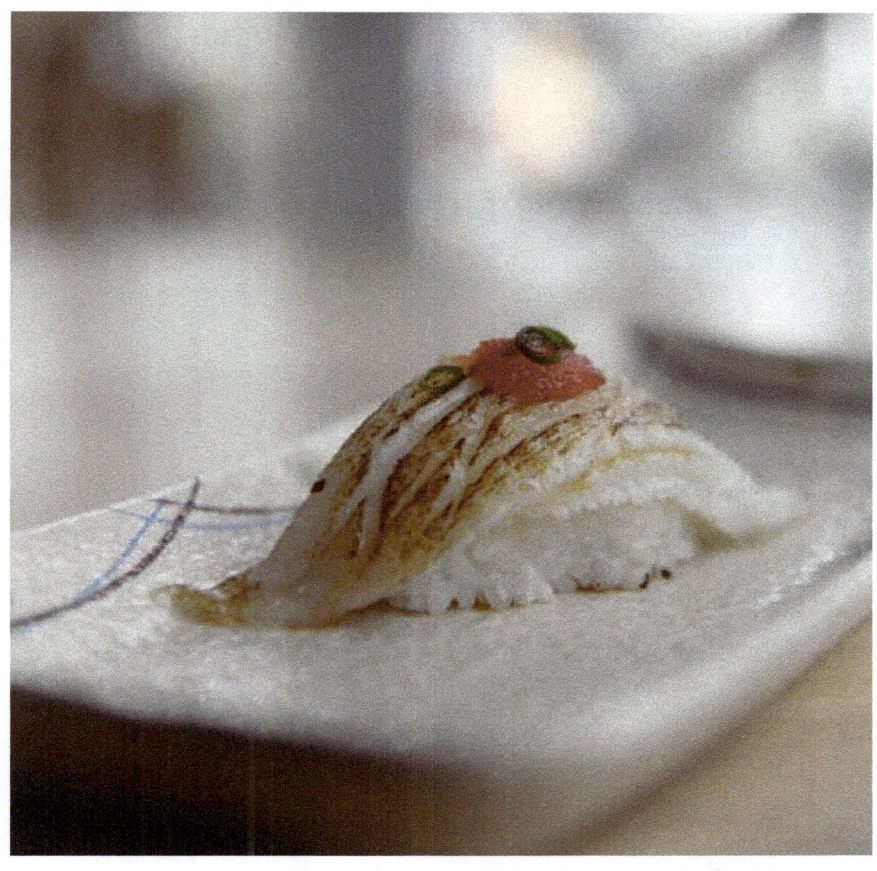

Preparation time: 30 minutes

Cooking time: 10 minutes

Servings: 3

Ingredients:
- 1 pound halibut steaks 2/3 cup soy sauce
  1/4 cup sugar
  2 tablespoons lime juice 1/2 cup mirin
- 1/4 teaspoon red pepper flakes, crushed 1/4 cup orange juice
- 1/4 teaspoon ginger, grated
- 1 garlic clove, minced

Directions:
√ Put soy sauce in a pan, heat up over medium heat, add mirin, sugar, lime and orange juice, pepper flakes, ginger and garlic, stir well, bring to a boil and take off heat.
√ Transfer half of the marinade to a bowl, add halibut, toss to coat and leave aside in the fridge for 30 minutes.
√ Transfer halibut to your air fryer and cook at 390 degrees F for 10 minutes, flipping once.
√ Divide halibut steaks on plates, drizzle the rest of the marinade all over and serve hot. Enjoy!

Nutrition: calories 286, fat 5, fiber 12, carbs 14, protein 23

Cod and Vinaigrette

Preparation time: 10 minutes

Cooking time: 15 minutes

Servings: 4

Ingredients:

- 4 cod fillets, skinless and boneless
- 12 cherry tomatoes, halved
- 8 black olives, pitted and roughly chopped 2 tablespoons lemon juice
- Salt and black pepper to the taste
- 2 tablespoons olive oil
- Cooking spray
- 1 bunch basil, chopped

Directions:

√ Season cod with salt and pepper to the taste, place in your air fryer's basket and cook at 360 degrees F for 10 minutes, flipping after 5 minutes.

√ Meanwhile, heat up a pan with the oil over medium heat, add tomatoes, olives and lemon juice, stir, bring to a simmer, add basil, salt and pepper, stir well and take off heat.

√   Divide fish on plates and serve with the vinaigrette drizzled on top.

Enjoy!

Nutrition: calories 300, fat 5, fiber 8, carbs 12, protein 8

Shrimp and Crab Mix

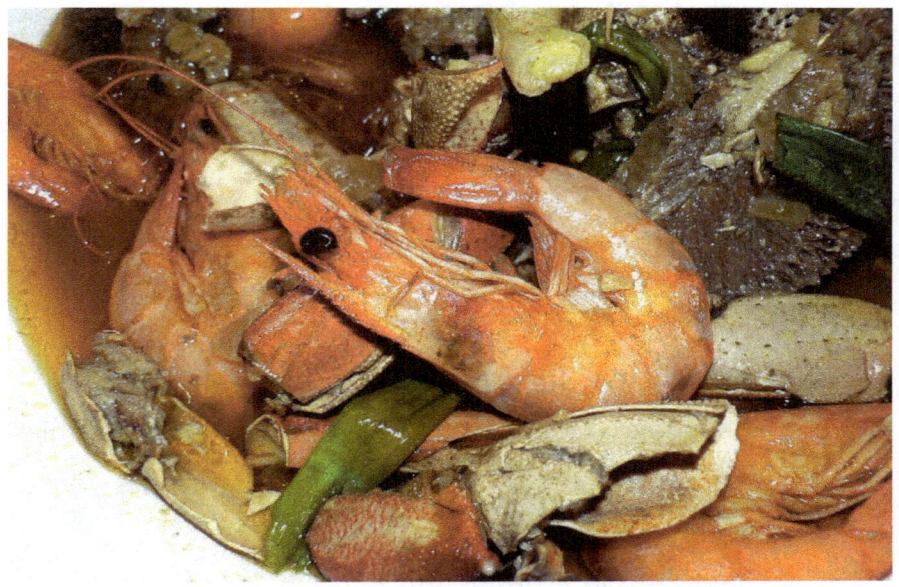

Preparation time: 10 minutes

Cooking time: 25 minutes

Servings: 4

Ingredients:

- 1/2 cup yellow onion, chopped
- 1 cup green bell pepper, chopped
- 1 cup celery, chopped

- 1 pound shrimp, peeled and deveined 1 cup crabmeat, flaked
- 1 cup mayonnaise
- 1 teaspoon Worcestershire sauce
- Salt and black pepper to the taste
- 2 tablespoons breadcrumbs
- 1 tablespoon butter, melted
- 1 teaspoon sweet paprika

Directions:

√ In a bowl, mix shrimp with crab meat, bell pepper, onion, mayo, celery, salt, pepper and Worcestershire sauce, toss well and transfer to a pan that fits your air fryer.

√ Sprinkle bread crumbs and paprika, add melted butter, place in your air fryer and cook at 320 degrees F for 25 minutes, shaking halfway.

√ Divide among plates and serve right away.

Enjoy!

Nutrition: calories 200, fat 13, fiber 9, carbs 17, protein 19

Seafood Casserole

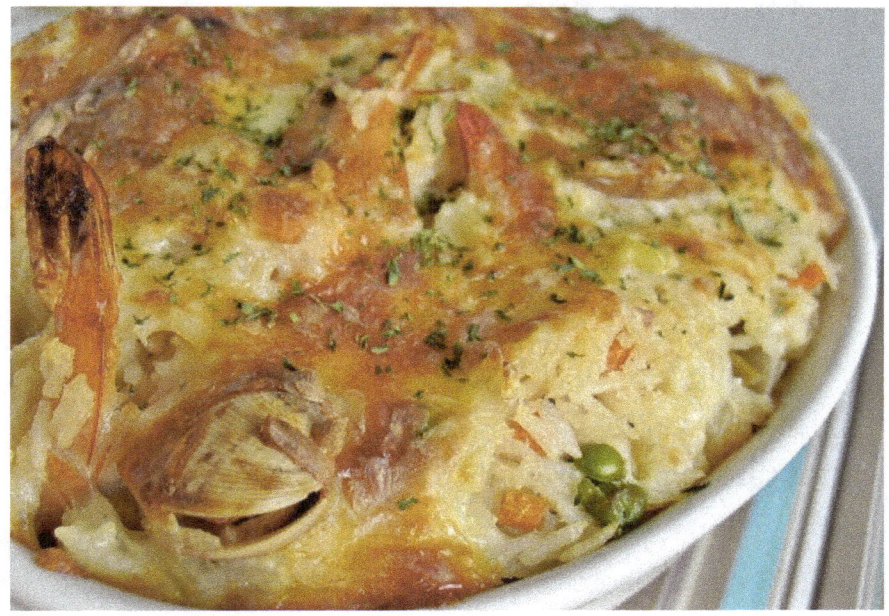

Preparation time: 10 minutes

Cooking time: 40 minutes

Servings: 6

Ingredients:

- 6 tablespoons butter
- 2 ounces mushrooms, chopped
- 1 small green bell pepper, chopped 1 celery stalk, Chopped

- 2 garlic cloves, mince
- 1 small yellow onion, chopped Salt and black pepper to the taste
- 4 tablespoons flour
- 1/2 cup white wine
- 1 and 1/2 cups milk
- 1/2 cup heavy cream
- 4 sea scallops, sliced
- 4 ounces haddock, skinless, boneless and cut into small pieces 4 ounces lobster meat, already cooked and cut into small pieces 1/2 teaspoon mustard powder
- 1 tablespoon lemon juice

- 1/3 cup bread crumbs
- Salt and black pepper to the taste
- 3 tablespoons cheddar cheese, grated A handful parsley, chopped
- 1 teaspoon sweet paprika

Directions:

√ Heat up a pan with 4 tablespoons butter over medium high heat, add bell pepper, mushrooms, celery, garlic, onion and wine, stir and cook for 10 minutes

√ Add flour, cream and milk, stir well and cook for 6 minutes.

Add lemon juice, salt, pepper, mustard powder, scallops, lobster meat and haddock, stir well, take off heat and transfer to a pan that fits your air fryer.
√ In a bowl, mix the rest of the butter with bread crumbs, paprika and cheese and sprinkle over seafood mix.
√ Transfer pan to your air fryer and cook at 360 degrees F for 16 minutes.
√ Divide among plates and serve with parsley sprinkled on top. Enjoy!

Nutrition: calories 270, fat 32, fiber 14, carbs 15, protein 23

Trout Fillet and Orange Sauce

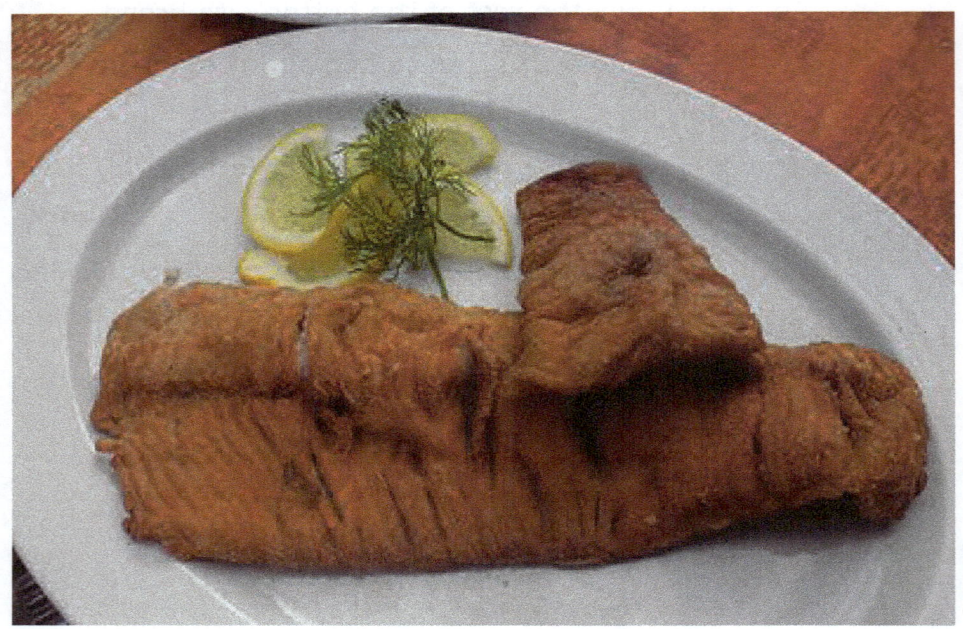

Preparation time: 10 minutes

Cooking time: 10 minutes

Servings: 4

Ingredients:

- 4 trout fillets, skinless and boneless 4 spring onions, chopped
- 1 tablespoon olive oil
- 1 tablespoon ginger, minced

- Salt and black pepper to the taste Juice and zest from 1 orange

Directions:

√ Season trout fillets with salt, pepper, rub them with the olive oil, place in a pan that fits your air fryer, add ginger, green onions, orange zest and juice, toss well, place in your air fryer and cook at 360 degrees F for 10 minutes.

√ Divide fish and sauce on plates and serve right away.

Enjoy!

Nutrition: calories 239, fat 10, fiber 7, carbs 18, protein 23

Cod Fillets and Peas

Preparation time: 10 minutes

Cooking time: 10 minutes

Servings: 4

Ingredients:

- 4 cod fillets, boneless
- 2 tablespoons parsley, chopped 2 cups peas
- 4 tablespoons wine
- 1/2 teaspoon oregano, dried
- 1/2 teaspoon sweet paprika
- 2 garlic cloves, minced
- Salt and pepper to the taste

Directions:

- √ In your food processor mix garlic with parsley, salt, pepper, oregano, paprika and wine and blend well.
- √ Rub fish with half of this mix, place in your air fryer and cook at 360 degrees F for 10 minutes.
- √ Meanwhile, put peas in a pot, add water to cover, add salt, bring to a boil over medium high

heat, cook for 10 minutes, drain and divide among plates.

√ Also divide fish on plates, spread the rest of the herb dressing all over and serve. Enjoy!

Nutrition: calories 261, fat 8, fiber 12, carbs 20, protein 22

Thyme and Parsley Salmon

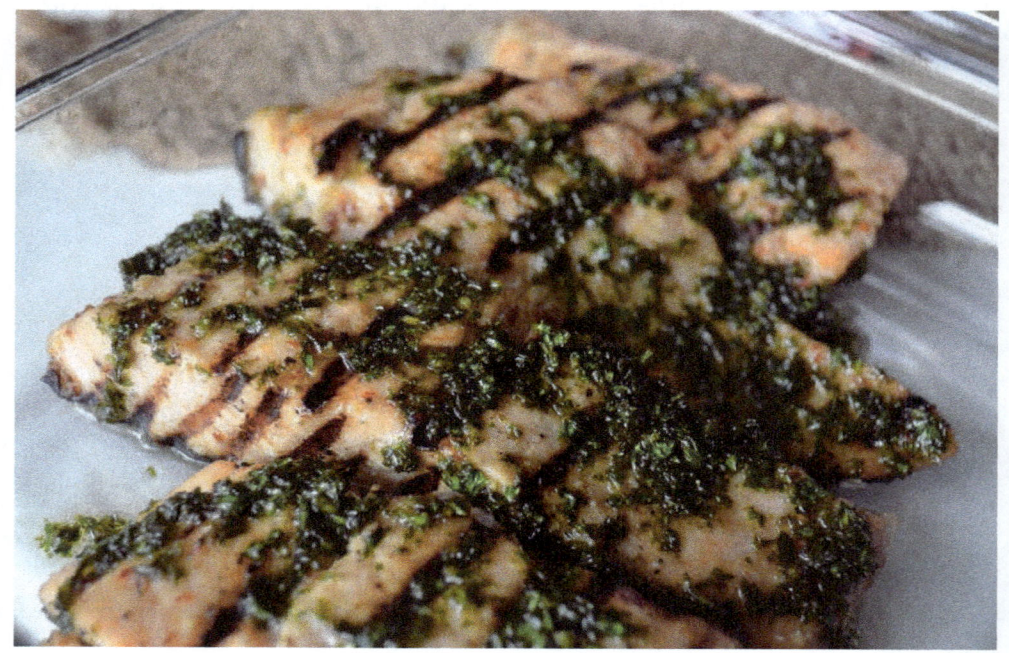

Preparation time: 10 minutes

Cooking time: 15 minutes

Servings: 4

Ingredients:

- 4 salmon fillets, boneless Juice from 1 lemon
- 1 yellow onion, chopped 3 tomatoes, sliced
- 4 thyme springs

- 4 parsley springs
- 3 tablespoons extra virgin olive oil Salt and black pepper to the taste

Directions:

√ Drizzle 1 tablespoon oil in a pan that fits your air fryer,, add a layer of tomatoes, salt and pepper, drizzle 1 more tablespoon oil, add fish, season them with salt and pepper, drizzle the rest of the oil, add thyme and parsley springs, onions, lemon juice, salt and pepper, place in your air fryer's basket and cook at 360 degrees F for 12 minutes shaking once.

√ Divide everything on plates and serve right away.

Enjoy!

Nutrition: calories 242, fat 9, fiber 12, carbs 20, protein 31

Trout and Butter Sauce

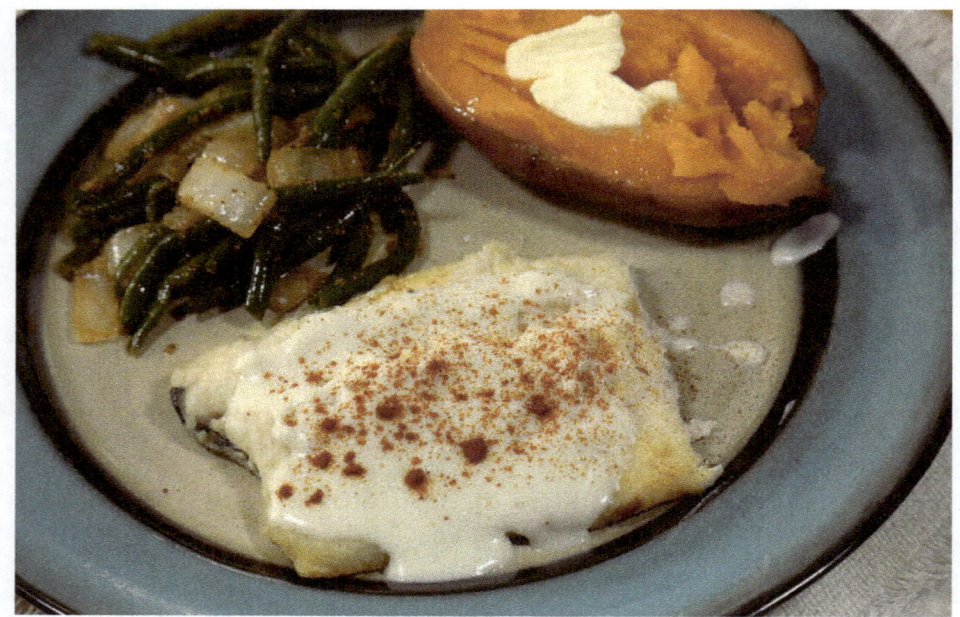

Preparation time: 10 minutes

Cooking time: 10 minutes

Servings: 4

Ingredients:

- 4 trout fillets, boneless
- Salt and black pepper to the taste 3 teaspoons
- lemon zest, grated
- 3 tablespoons chives, chopped

- 6 tablespoons butter
- 2 tablespoons olive oil
- 2 teaspoons lemon juice

Directions:

- √ Season trout with salt and pepper, drizzle the olive oil, rub, transfer to your air fryer and cook at 360 degrees F for 10 minutes, flipping once.
- √ Meanwhile, heat up a pan with the butter over medium heat, add salt, pepper, chives, lemon juice and zest, whisk well, cook for 1-2 minutes and take off heat
- √ Divide fish fillets on plates, drizzle butter sauce all over and serve.

Enjoy!

Nutrition: calories 300, fat 12, fiber 9, carbs 27, protein 24

Creamy Salmon

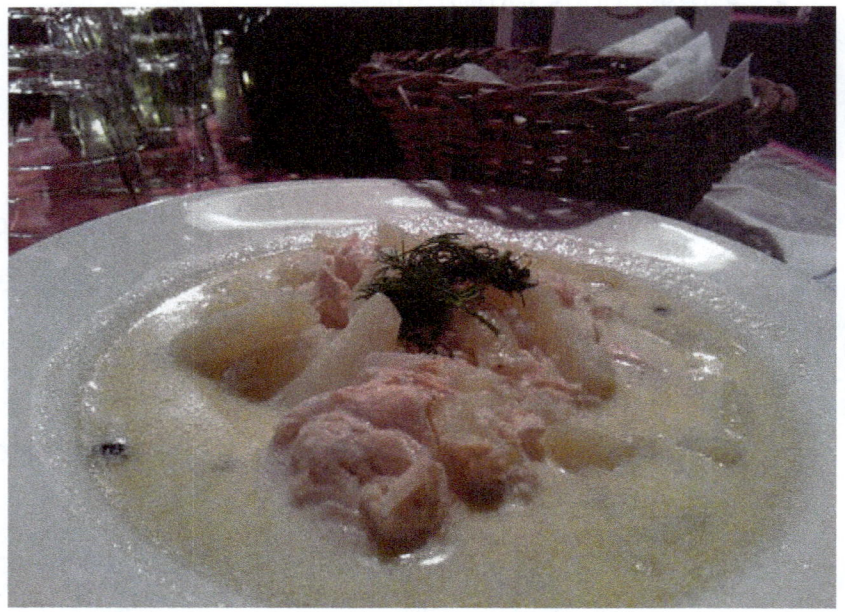

Preparation time: 10 minutes

Cooking time: 10 minutes

Servings: 4

Ingredients:

- 4 salmon fillets, boneless
- 1 tablespoons olive oil
- Salt and black pepper to the taste 1/3 cup cheddar cheese, grated

- 1 and 1/2 teaspoon mustard
- 1/2 cup coconut cream

Directions:

√ Season salmon with salt and pepper, drizzle the oil and rub well.
√ In a bowl, mix coconut cream with cheddar, mustard, salt and pepper and stir well.
√ Transfer salmon to a pan that fits your air fryer, add coconut cream mix, introduce in your air fryer and cook at 320 degrees F for 10 minutes.
√ Divide among plates and serve.

Enjoy!

Nutrition: calories 200, fat 6, fiber 14, carbs 17, protein 20

Salmon & Avocado Salsa

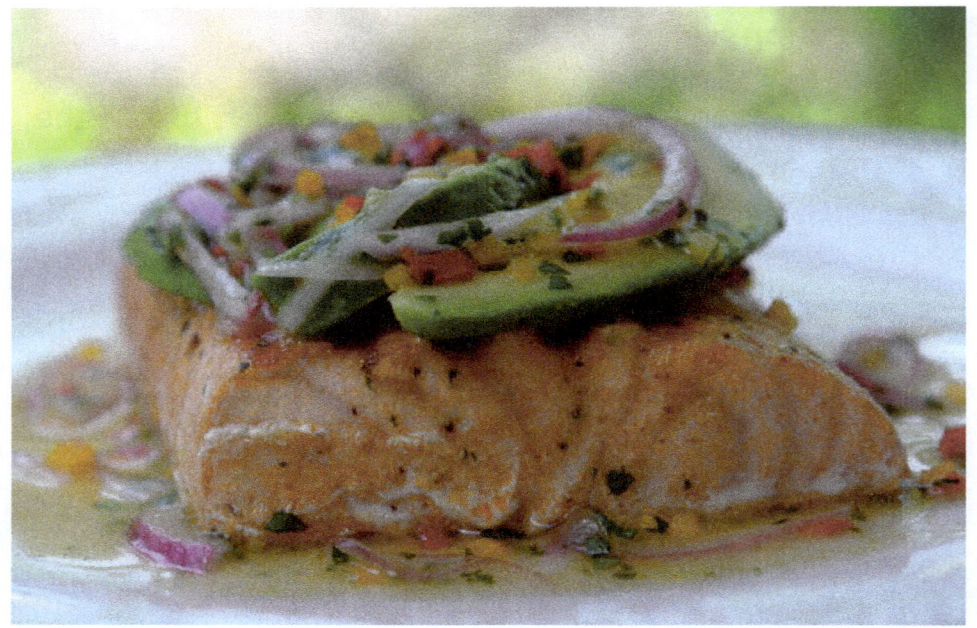

Preparation time: 30 minutes

Cooking time: 10 minutes

Servings: 4

Ingredients:

- 4 salmon fillets
- 1 tablespoon olive oil

- Salt and black pepper to the taste 1 teaspoon cumin, ground
- 1 teaspoon sweet paprika
- 1/2 teaspoon chili powder
- 1 teaspoon garlic powder
- *For the salsa:*
- 1 small red onion, chopped
- 1 avocado, pitted,
- peeled and chopped 2 tablespoons cilantro, chopped
- Juice from 2 limes
- Salt and black pepper to the taste

Directions:

- √ In a bowl, mix salt, pepper, chili powder, onion powder, paprika and cumin, stir, rub salmon with this mix, drizzle the oil, rub again, transfer to your air fryer and cook at 350 degrees F for 5 minutes on each side.
- √ Meanwhile, in a bowl, mix avocado with red onion, salt, pepper, cilantro and lime juice and stir.
- √ Divide fillets on plates, top with avocado salsa and serve.

Enjoy!

Nutrition: calories 300, fat 14, fiber 4, carbs 18, protein 16

Italian Barramundi Fillets and Tomato Salsa

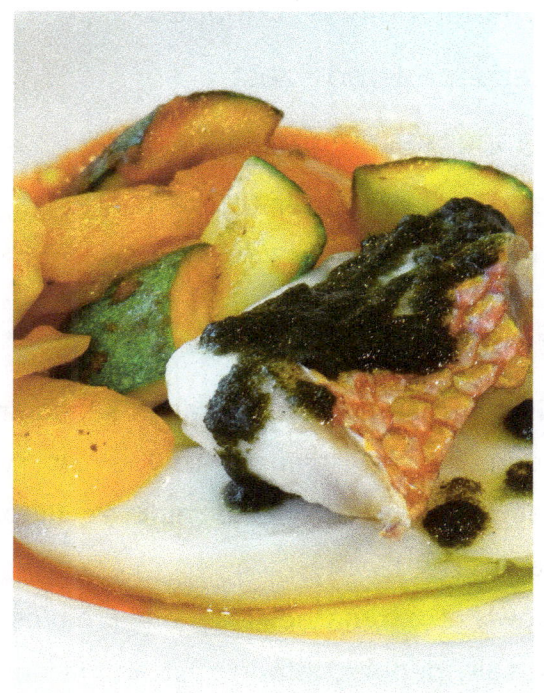

Preparation time: 10 minutes

Cooking time: 8 minutes

Servings: 4

Ingredients:

- 2 barramundi fillets, boneless
- 1 tablespoon olive oil+ 2 teaspoons

- 2 teaspoons Italian seasoning
- 1/4 cup green olives, pitted and chopped 1/4 cup
- cherry tomatoes, chopped
- 1/4 cup black olives, chopped
- 1 tablespoon lemon zest
- 2 tablespoons lemon zest
- Salt and black pepper to the taste
- 2 tablespoons parsley, chopped

Directions:

- Rub fish with salt, pepper, Italian seasoning and 2 teaspoons olive oil, transfer to your air fryer and cook at 360 degrees F for 8 minutes, flipping them halfway.
- In a bowl, mix tomatoes with black olives, green olives, salt, pepper, lemon zest and lemon juice, parsley and 1 tablespoon olive oil and toss well
- Divide fish on plates, add tomato salsa on top and serve. Enjoy!

Nutrition: calories 270, fat 4, fiber 2, carbs 18, protein 27

Creamy Shrimp and Veggies

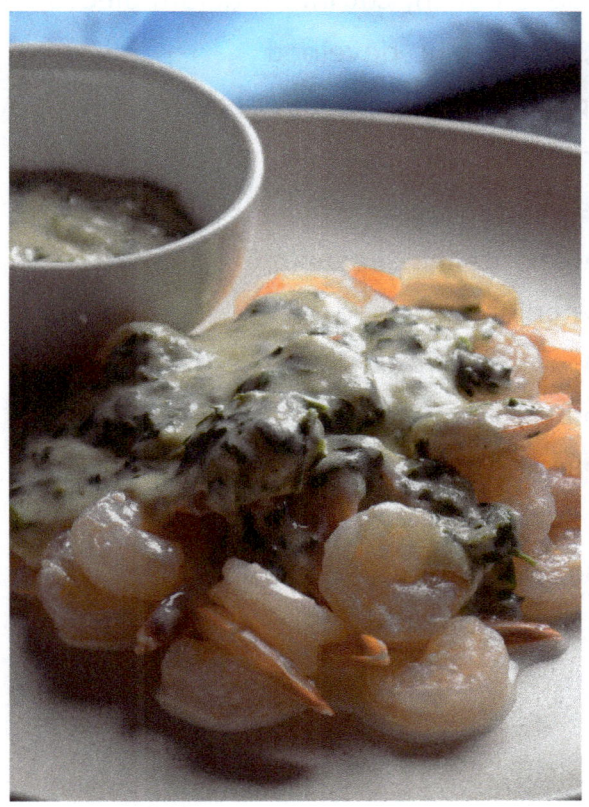

Preparation time: 10 minutes

Cooking time: 30 minutes

Servings: 4

Ingredients:

- 8 ounces mushrooms, chopped
- 1 asparagus bunch, cut into medium pieces 1 pound shrimp, peeled and deveined
- Salt and black pepper to the taste
- 1 spaghetti squash, cut into halves
- 2 tablespoons olive oil
- 2 teaspoons Italian seasoning
- 1 yellow onion, chopped
- 1 teaspoon red pepper flakes, crushed
- 1/4 cup butter, melted
- 1 cup parmesan cheese, grated
- 2 garlic cloves, minced
- 1 cup heavy cream

Directions:

√ Place squash halves in you air fryer's basket, cook at 390 degrees F for 17 minutes, transfer to a cutting board, scoop insides and transfer to a bowl.
√ Put water in a pot, add some salt, bring to a boil over medium heat, add asparagus, steam for a couple of minutes, transfer to a bowl filled with ice water, drain and leave aside as well.

- √ Heat up a pan that fits your air fryer with the oil over medium heat, add onions and mushrooms, stir and cook for 7 minutes.
- √ Add pepper flakes, Italian seasoning, salt, pepper, squash, asparagus, shrimp, melted butter, cream, parmesan and garlic, toss and cook in your air fryer at 360 degrees F for 6 minutes.

  Divide everything on plates and serve.

Enjoy!

Nutrition: calories 325, fat 6, fiber 5, carbs 14, protein 13

Stuffed Calamari

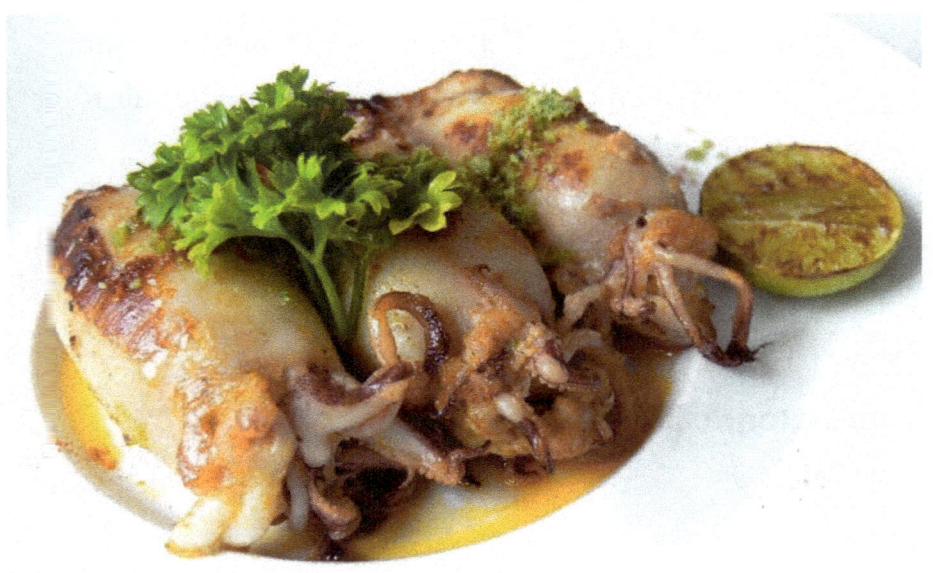

Preparation time: 10 minutes

Cooking time: 25 minutes

Servings: 4

Ingredients:

- 4 big calamari, tentacles separated and chopped and tubes reserved 2 tablespoons parsley, chopped
- 5 ounces kale, chopped

- 2 garlic cloves, minced
- 1 red bell pepper, chopped
- 1 tablespoon olive oil
- 2 ounces canned tomato puree
- 1 yellow onion, chopped
- Salt and black pepper to the taste

Directions:

1. Heat up a pan with the oil over medium heat, add onion and garlic, stir and cook for 2 minutes.
2. Add bell pepper, tomato puree, calamari tentacles, kale, salt and pepper, stir, cook for 10 minutes and take off heat. stir and cook for 3 minutes.
3. Stuff calamari tubes with this mix, secure with toothpicks, put in your air fryer and cook at 360 degrees F for 20 minutes.
   Divide calamari on plates, sprinkle parsley all over and serve.

Enjoy!

Nutrition: calories 322, fat 10, fiber 14, carbs 14, protein 22

Salmon and Chives Vinaigrette

Preparation time: 10 minutes

Cooking time: 12 minutes

Servings: 4

Ingredients:

- 2 tablespoons dill, chopped
- 4 salmon fillets, boneless
- 2 tablespoons chives, chopped 1/3 cup maple syru
- 1 tablespoon olive oil
- 3 tablespoons balsamic vinegar Salt and black pepper to the taste

Directions:

1. Season fish with salt and pepper, rub with the oil, place in your air fryer and cook at 350 degrees F for 8 minutes, flipping once.
2. Heat up a small pot with the vinegar over medium heat, add maple syrup, chives and dill, stir and cook for 3 minutes.
3. Divide fish on plates and serve with chives vinaigrette on top.

Enjoy!

Nutrition: calories 270, fat 3, fiber 13, carbs 25, protein 10

Halibut and Sun Dried Tomatoes Mix

Preparation time: 10 minutes

Cooking time: 10 minutes

Servings: 2

Ingredients:

- 2 medium halibut fillets
- 2 garlic cloves, minced
- 2 teaspoons olive oil
- Salt and black pepper to the taste 6 sun dried tomatoes, chopped
- 2 small red onions, sliced
- 1 fennel bulb, sliced
- 9 black olives, pitted and sliced
- 4 rosemary springs, chopped
- ½ teaspoon red pepper flakes, crushed

Directions:

1. Season fish with salt, pepper, rub with garlic and oil and put in a heat proof dish that fits your air fryer.
2. Add onion slices, sun dried tomatoes, fennel, olives, rosemary and sprinkle pepper flakes, transfer to your air fryer and cook at 380 degrees F for 10 minutes.

3. Divide fish and veggies on plates and serve.

Enjoy!

Nutrition: calories 300, fat 12, fiber 9, carbs 18, protein 30

Black Cod and Plum Sauce

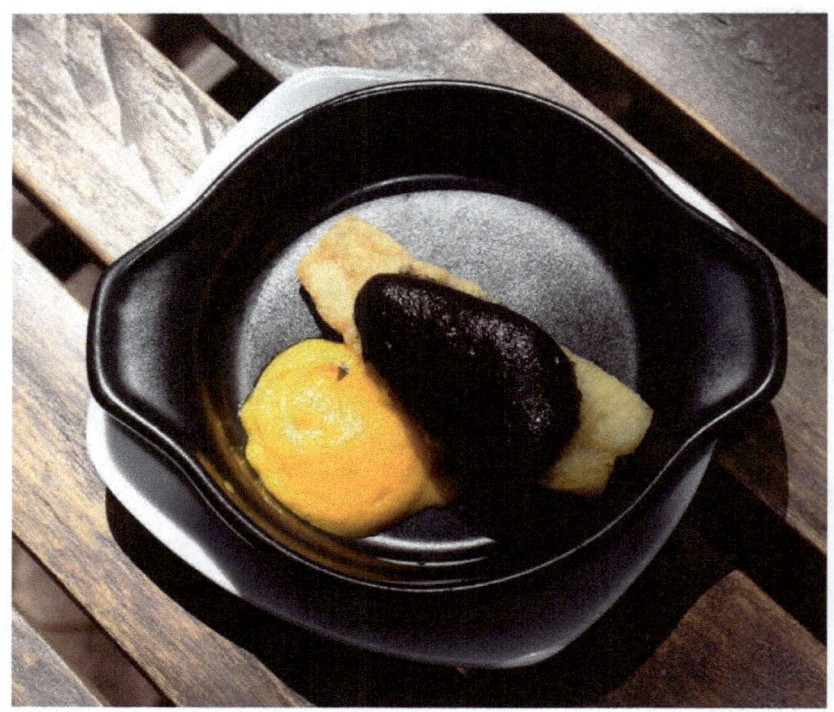

Preparation time: 10 minutes

Cooking time: 15 minutes

Servings: 2

Ingredients:

- 1 egg white

- ½ cup red quinoa, already cooked
- 2 teaspoons whole wheat flour
- 4 teaspoons lemon juice
- ½ teaspoon smoked paprika
- 1 teaspoon olive oil
- 2 medium black cod fillets, skinless and boneless 1 red plum, pitted and chopped
- 2 teaspoons raw honey
- ¼ teaspoon black peppercorns, crushed
- 2 teaspoons parsley
- ¼ cup water

Directions:

1. In a bowl, mix 1 teaspoon lemon juice with egg white, flour and ¼ teaspoon paprika and whisk well.
2. Put quinoa in a bowl and mix it with 1/3 of egg white mix.
   Put the fish into the bowl with the remaining egg white mix and toss to coat.
3. Dip fish in quinoa mix, coat well and leave aside for 10 minutes.
4. Heat up a pan with 1 teaspoon oil over medium heat, add peppercorns, honey and plum, stir, bring to a simmer and cook for 1 minute.

5. Add the rest of the lemon juice, the rest of the paprika and the water, stir well and simmer for 5 minutes.
6. Add parsley, stir, take sauce off heat and leave aside for now.
    Put fish in your air fryer and cook at 380 degrees F for 10 minutes Arrange fish on plates, drizzle plum sauce on top and serve.

Enjoy!

Nutrition: calories 324, fat 14, fiber 22, carbs 27, protein 22

Fish and Couscous

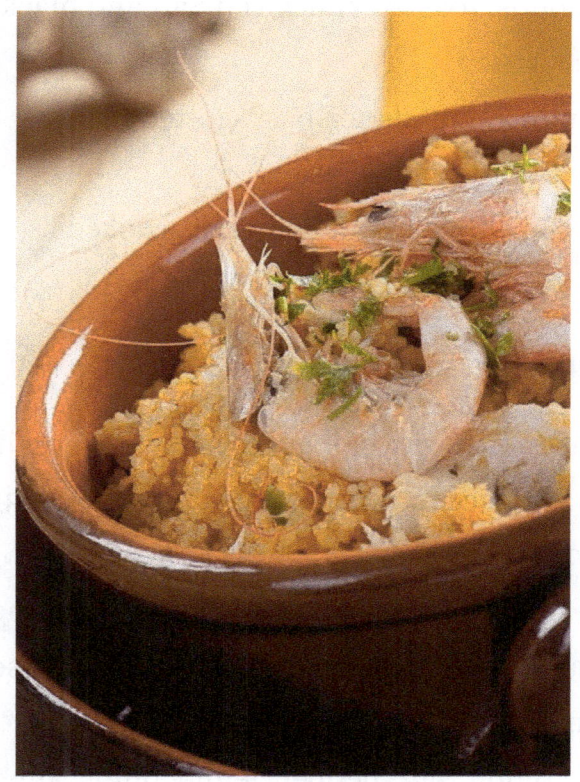

Preparation time: 10 minutes

Cooking time: 15 minutes

Servings: 4

Ingredients:

- 2 red onions, chopped

- Cooking spray
- 2 small fennel bulbs, cored and sliced 1/4 cup
- almonds, toasted and sliced Salt and black pepper to the taste
- 2 and 1/2 pounds sea bass, gutted
- 5 teaspoons fennel seeds
- 3/4 cup whole wheat couscous, cooked

Directions:

1. Season fish with salt and pepper, spray with cooking spray, place in your air fryer and cook at 350 degrees F for 10 minutes.
2. Meanwhile, spray a pan with some cooking oil and heat it up over medium heat. Add fennel seeds to this pan, stir and toast them for 1 minute.
3. Add onion, salt, pepper, fennel bulbs, almonds and couscous, stir, cook for 2-3 minutes and divide among plates.
Add fish next to couscous mix and serve right away. Enjoy!

Nutrition: calories 354, fat 7, fiber 10, carbs 20, protein 30

Chinese Cod

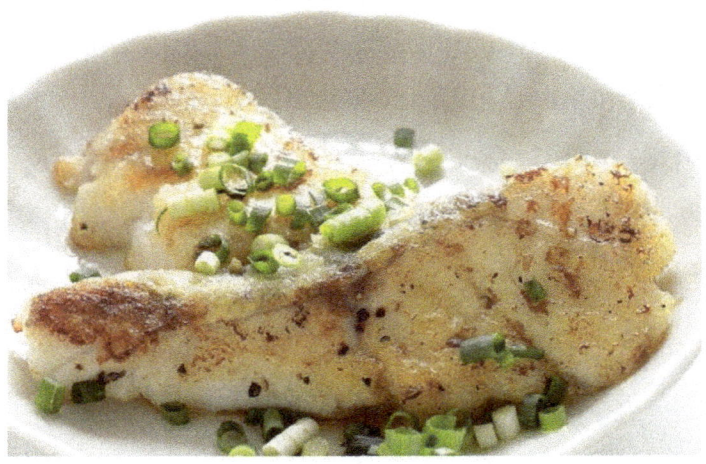

Preparation time: 10 minutes

Cooking time: 10 minutes

Servings: 2

Ingredients:

- 2 medium cod fillets, boneless 1 teaspoon peanuts, crushed
- 2 teaspoons garlic powder
- 1 tablespoon light soy sauce ½ teaspoon ginger, grated

Directions:

1. Put fish fillets in a heat proof dish that fits your air fryer, add garlic powder, soy sauce and ginger, toss well, put in your air fryer and cook at 350 degrees F for 10 minutes.
2. Divide fish on plates, sprinkle peanuts on top and serve.

Enjoy!

Nutrition: calories 254, fat 10, fiber 11, carbs 14, protein 23

Cod with Pearl Onions

Preparation time: 10 minutes

Cooking time: 15 minutes

Servings: 2

Ingredients:

- 14 ounces pearl onions
- 2 medium cod fillets
- 1 tablespoon parsley, dried 1 teaspoon thyme, dried
- Black pepper to the taste
- 8 ounces mushrooms, sliced

Directions:

1. Put fish in a heat proof dish that fits your air fryer,
2. Add onions, parsley, mushrooms, thyme and black pepper, toss well,
3. Put in your air fryer and cook at 350 degrees F and cook for 15 minutes.
4. Divide everything on plates and serve.

Enjoy!

Nutrition: calories 270, fat 14, fiber 8, carbs 14, protein 22

Hawaiian Salmon

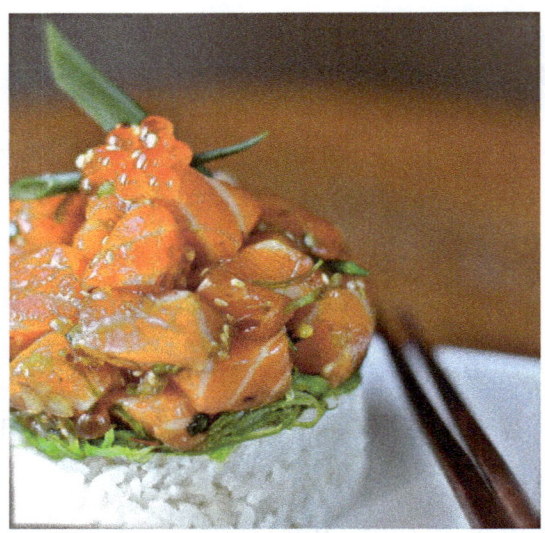

Preparation time: 10 minutes

Cooking time: 10 minutes

Servings: 2

Ingredients:

- 20 ounces canned pineapple pieces and juice ½ teaspoon ginger, grated
- 2 teaspoons garlic powder
- 1 teaspoon onion powder
- 1 tablespoon balsamic vinegar

- 2 medium salmon fillets, boneless Salt and black pepper to the taste

Directions:

1. Season salmon with garlic powder, onion powder, salt and black pepper, rub well, transfer to a heat proof dish that fits your air fryer, add ginger and pineapple chunks and toss them really gently.
2. Drizzle the vinegar all over, put in your air fryer and cook at 350 degrees F for 10 minutes.
3. Divide everything on plates and serve..
4. Enjoy!

    Nutrition: calories 200, fat 8, fiber 12, carbs 17, protein 20

Salmon and Avocado Salad

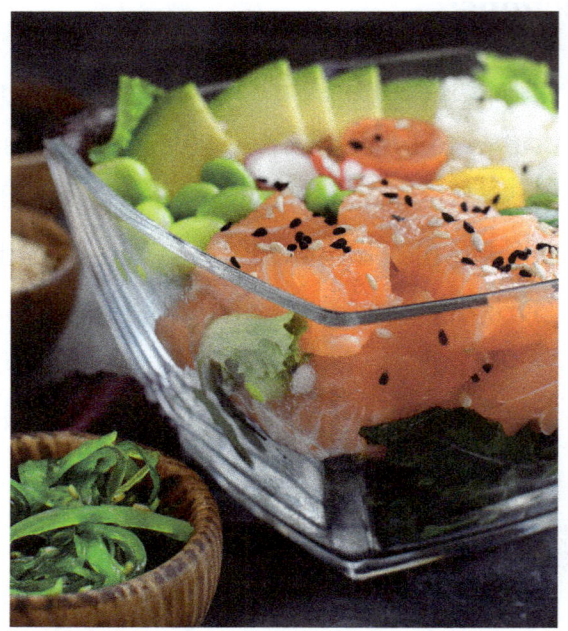

Preparation time: 10 minutes

Cooking time: 20 minutes

 Servings: 4

Ingredients:

- 2 medium salmon fillets
- ¼ cup melted butter
- 4 ounces mushrooms, sliced

- Sea salt and black pepper to the taste 12 cherry tomatoes, halved
- 2 tablespoons olive oil
- 8 ounces lettuce leaves, torn
- 1 avocado, pitted, peeled and cubed 1 jalapeno
- pepper, chopped
- 5 cilantro springs, chopped
- 2 tablespoons white wine vinegar
- 1 ounce feta cheese, crumbled

Directions:

1. Place salmon on a lined baking sheet, brush with 2 tablespoons melted butter, season with salt and pepper, broil for 15 minutes over medium heat and then keep warm.
2. Meanwhile, heat up a pan with the rest of the butter over medium heat, add mushrooms, stir and cook for a few minutes.
3. Put tomatoes in a bowl, add salt, pepper and 1 tablespoon olive oil and toss to coat.
4. In a salad bowl, mix salmon with mushrooms, lettuce, avocado, tomatoes, jalapeno and cilantro.
5. Add the rest of the oil, vinegar, salt and pepper, sprinkle cheese on top and serve. Enjoy!

Nutrition: calories 235, fat 6, fiber 8, carbs 19, protein 5

Salmon and Greek Yogurt Sauce

Preparation time: 10 minutes

Cooking time: 20 minutes

Servings: 2

Ingredients:

- 2 medium salmon fillets
- 1 tablespoon basil, chopped
- 6 lemon slices
- Sea salt and black pepper to the taste 1 cup Greek yogurt
- 2 teaspoons curry powder
- A pinch of cayenne pepper
- 1 garlic clove, minced
- ½ teaspoon cilantro, chopped
- ½ teaspoon mint, chopped

Directions:

1. Place each salmon fillet on a parchment paper piece, make 3 splits in each and stuff them with basil.
2. Season with salt and pepper, top each fillet with 3 lemon slices, fold parchment, seal edges, introduce in the oven at 400 degrees F and bake for 20 minutes.

3. Meanwhile, in a bowl, mix yogurt with cayenne pepper, salt to the taste, garlic, curry, mint and cilantro and whisk well.
4. Transfer fish to plates, drizzle the yogurt sauce you've just prepared on top and serve right away! Enjoy!

Nutrition: calories 242, fat 1, fiber 2, carbs 3, protein 3

Special Salmon

Preparation time: 10 minutes

Cooking time: 25 minutes

Servings: 4

Ingredients:

- 1 pound medium beets, sliced 6 tablespoons olive oil
- 1 and 1/2 pounds salmon fillets, skinless and boneless
- Salt and pepper to the taste
- 1 tablespoon chives, chopped
- 1 tablespoon parsley, chopped
- 1 tablespoon fresh tarragon, chopped 3 tablespoon shallots, chopped
- 1 tablespoon grated lemon zest
- 1/4 cup lemon juice
- 4 cups mixed baby greens

Directions:

1. In a bowl, mix beets with 1/2 tablespoon oil and toss to coat.
   Season them with salt and pepper, arrange them on a baking sheet, introduce in
2. the oven at 450 degrees F and bake for 20 minutes.

3. Take beets out of the oven, add salmon on top, brush it with the rest if the oil and season with salt and pepper.
4. In a bowl, mix chives with parsley and tarragon and sprinkle 1 tablespoon of this mix over salmon.
5. Introduce in the oven again and bake for 15 minutes. Meanwhile, in a boil with shallots with lemon peel, salt, pepper and lemon juice and the rest of the herbs mixture and stir gently.
6. Combine 2 tablespoons of shallots dressing with mixed greens and toss gently.
7. Take salmon out of the oven, arrange on plates, add beets and greens on the side, drizzle the rest of the shallot dressing on top and serve right away.

Enjoy!

Nutrition: calories 312, fat 2, fiber 2, carbs 2, protein 4

Spanish Salmon

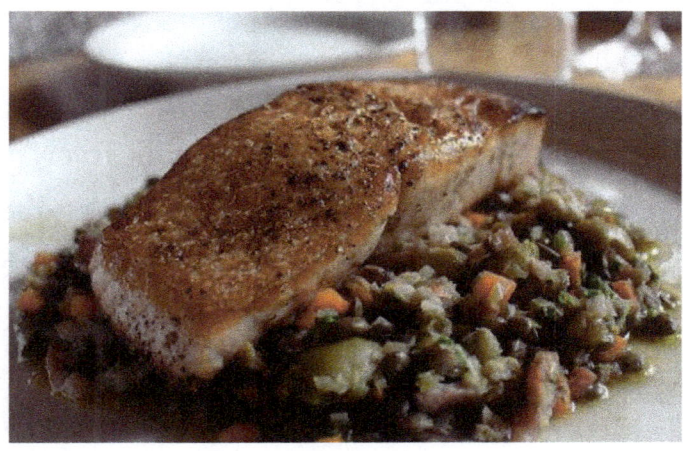

Preparation time: 10 minutes

Cooking time: 15 minutes

Servings: 6

Ingredients:

- 2 cups bread crouton
- 3 red onions, cut into medium wedges ¾ cup green olives, pitted
- 3 red bell peppers, cut into medium wedges ½ teaspoon smoked paprika Salt and black pepper to the taste

- 5 tablespoons olive oil
- 6 medium salmon fillets, skinless and boneless 2 tablespoons parsley, chopped

Directions:

1. In a heat proof dish that fits your air fryer, mix bread croutons with onion wedges, bell pepper ones, olives, salt, pepper, paprika and 3 tablespoons olive oil, toss well, place in your air fryer and cook at 356 degrees F for 7 minutes.
2. Rub salmon with the rest of the oil, add over veggies and cook at 360 degrees F for 8 minutes.
3. Divide fish and veggie mix on plates, sprinkle parsley all over and serve.

Enjoy!

Nutrition: calories 321, fat 8, fiber 14, carbs 27, protein 22

Marinated Salmon

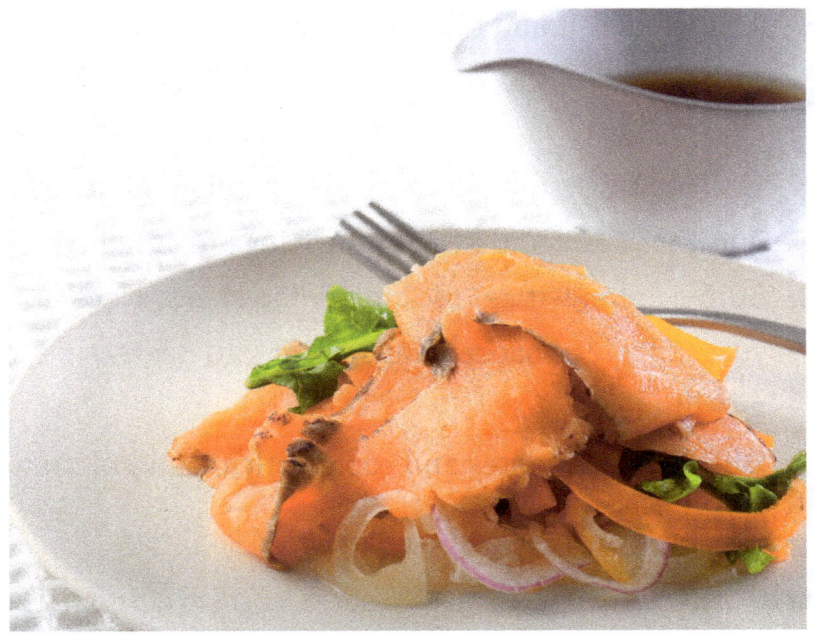

Preparation time: 1 hour

Cooking time: 20 minutes

Servings: 6

Ingredients:

- 1 whole salmon
- 1 tablespoon dill, chopped

- 1 tablespoon tarragon, chopped 1 tablespoon garlic, minced Juice from 2 lemons
- 1 lemon, sliced
- A pinch of salt and black pepper

Directions:

1. In a large fish, mix fish with salt, pepper and lemon juice, toss well and keep in the fridge for 1 hour.
2. Stuff salmon with garlic and lemon slices, place in your air fryer's basket and cook at 320 degrees F for 25 minutes.
3. Divide among plates and serve with a tasty coleslaw on the side. Enjoy!

Nutrition: calories 300, fat 8, fiber 9, carbs 19, protein 27

Delicious Red Snapper

Preparation time: 30 minutes

Cooking time: 15 minutes

Servings: 4

Ingredients:

- 1 big red snapper, cleaned and scored Salt
- black pepper to the taste
- 3 garlic cloves, minced
- 1 jalapeno, chopped
- 1/4 pound okra, chopped
- 1 tablespoon butter
- 2 tablespoons olive oil
- 1 red bell pepper, chopped
- 2 tablespoons white wine
- 2 tablespoons parsley, chopped

Directions:

1. In a bowl, mix jalapeno, wine with garlic, stir well and rub snapper with this mix.
2. Season fish with salt and pepper and leave it aside for 30 minutes.
   Meanwhile, heat up a pan with 1 tablespoon butter

over medium heat, add bell pepper and okra, stir and cook for 5 minutes.
3. Stuff red snapper's belly with this mix, also add parsley and rub with the olive oil.
4. Place in preheated air fryer and cook at 400 degrees F for 15 minutes, flipping the fish halfway.
5. Divide among plates and serve. Enjoy!

Nutrition: calories 261, fat 7, fiber 18, carbs 28, protein 18

Snapper Fillets and Veggies

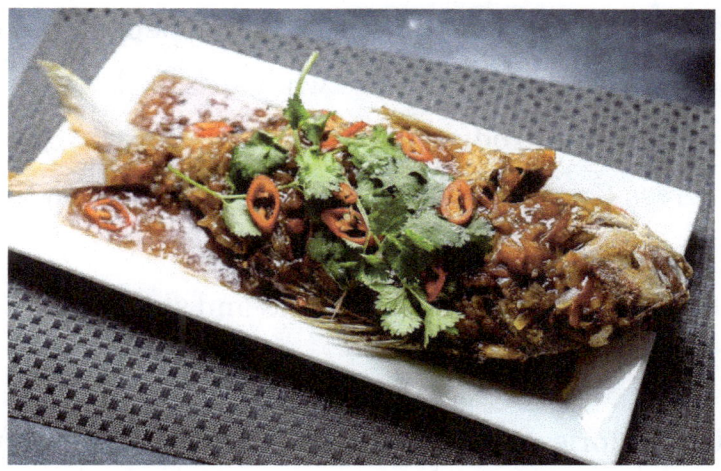

Preparation time: 10 minutes

Cooking time: 14 minutes

Servings: 2

Ingredients:

- 2 red snapper fillets, boneless
- 1 tablespoon olive oil
- ½ cup red bell pepper, chopped ½ cup green bell pepper, chopped ½ cup leeks, chopped
- Salt and black pepper to the taste 1 teaspoon
- tarragon, dried
- A splash of white wine

Directions:

1. In a heat proof dish that fits your air fryer, mix fish fillets with salt, pepper, oil, green bell pepper, red bell pepper, leeks, tarragon and wine, toss well everything, introduce in preheated air fryer at 350 degrees F and cook for 14 minutes, flipping fish fillets halfway.
2. Divide fish and veggies on plates and serve warm. Enjoy!

Nutrition: calories 300, fat 12, fiber 8, carbs 29, protein 12

Air Fried Branzino

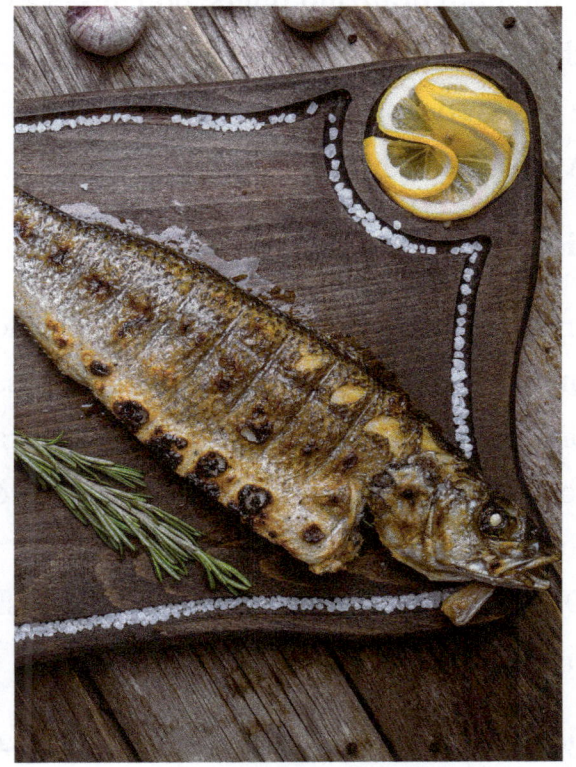

Preparation time: 10 minutes

Cooking time: 10 minutes

Servings: 4

Ingredients:

- Zest from 1 lemon, grated Zest from 1 orange, grated
- Juice from ½ lemon

- Juice from ½ orange
- Salt and black pepper to the taste
- 4 medium branzino fillets, boneless ½ cup parsley, chopped
- 2 tablespoons olive oil
- A pinch of red pepper flakes, crushed

Directions:

1. In a large bowl, mix fish fillets with lemon zest, orange zest, lemon juice, orange juice, salt, pepper, oil and pepper flakes, toss really well, transfer fillets to your preheated air fryer at 350 degrees F and bake for 10 minutes, flipping fillets once.
2. Divide fish on plates, sprinkle with parsley and serve right away. Enjoy!

Nutrition: calories 261, fat 8, fiber 12, carbs 21, protein 12

Lemon Sole and Swiss Chard

Preparation time: 10 minutes

Cooking time: 14 minutes

Servings: 4

Ingredients:

- 1 teaspoon lemon zest, grated 4 white bread slices, quartered 1/4 cup walnuts, chopped
- 1/4 cup parmesan, grated
- 4 tablespoons olive oil
- 4 sole fillets, boneless
- Salt and black pepper to the taste 4 tablespoons butter
- 1/4 cup lemon juice
- 3 tablespoons capers
- 2 garlic cloves, minced
- 2 bunches Swiss chard, chopped

Directions:

1. In your food processor, mix bread with walnuts, cheese and lemon zest and pulse well. Add half of the olive oil, pulse really well again and leave aside for now.

2. Heat up a pan with the butter over medium heat, add lemon juice, salt, pepper and capers, stir well, add fish and toss it.
3. Transfer fish to your preheated air fryer's basket, top with bread mix you've made at the beginning and cook at 350 degrees F for 14 minutes.
4. Meanwhile, heat up another pan with the rest of the oil, add garlic, Swiss chard, salt and pepper, stir gently, cook for 2 minutes and take off heat.
5. Divide fish on plates and serve with sautéed chard on the side.

Enjoy!

Nutrition: calories 321, fat 7, fiber 18, carbs 27, protein 12

Salmon and Blackberry Glaze

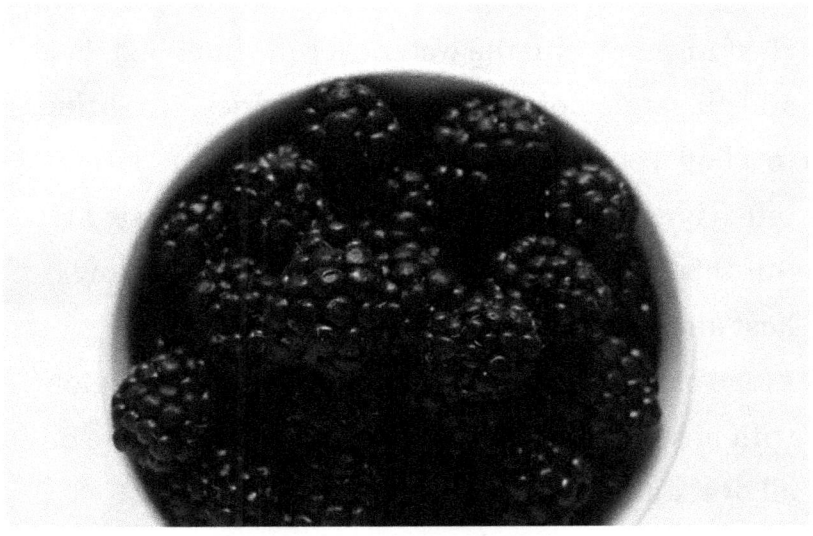

Preparation time: 10 minutes

Cooking time: 33 minutes

Servings: 4 Ingredients:

- 1 cup water
- 1 inch ginger piece, grated
- Juice from 1/2 lemon
- 12 ounces blackberries
- 1 tablespoon olive oil
- 1/4 cup sugar
- 4 medium salmon fillets, skinless Salt

- black pepper to the taste

Directions:

1. Heat up a pot with the water over medium high heat, add ginger, lemon juice and blackberries, stir, bring to a boil, cook for 4-5 minutes, take off heat, strain into a bowl, return to pan and combine with sugar. Stir this mix, bring to a simmer over medium low heat and cook for 20 minutes.
2. Leave blackberry sauce to cool down, brush salmon with it, season with salt and pepper, drizzle olive oil all over and rub fish well.
3. Place fish in your preheated air fryer at 350 degrees F and cook for 10 minutes, flipping fish fillets once.
4. Divide among plates, drizzle some of the remaining blackberry sauce all over and serve. Enjoy!

Nutrition: calories 312, fat 4, fiber 9, carbs 19, protein 14

Oriental Fish

Preparation time: 10 minutes

Cooking time: 12 minutes

Servings: 4

Ingredients:

- 2 pounds red snapper fillets, boneless Salt
- black pepper to the taste
- 3 garlic cloves, minced
- 1 yellow onion, chopped
- 1 tablespoon tamarind paste
- 1 tablespoon oriental sesame oil 1 tablespoon ginger, grated
- 2 tablespoons water
- 1/2 teaspoon cumin, ground
- 1 tablespoon lemon juice
- 3 tablespoons mint, chopped

Directions:

1. In your food processor, mix garlic with onion, salt, pepper, tamarind paste, sesame oil, ginger, water and cumin, pulse well and rub fish with this mix.
2. Place fish in your preheated air fryer at 320 degrees F and cook for 12 minutes, flipping fish halfway.

3. Divide fish on plates, drizzle lemon juice all over, sprinkle mint and serve right away. Enjoy!

Nutrition: calories 241, fat 8, fiber 16, carbs 17, protein 12

Delicious French Cod

Preparation time: 10 minutes

Cooking time: 22 minutes

Servings: 4

Ingredients:

- 2 tablespoons olive oil
- 1 yellow onion, chopped
- 1/2 cup white wine
- 2 garlic cloves, minced
- 14 ounces canned tomatoes,
- stewed 3 tablespoons parsley, chopped
- 2 pounds cod, boneless
- Salt and black pepper to the taste
- 2 tablespoons butter

Directions:

1. Heat up a pan with the oil over medium heat, add garlic and onion, stir and cook for 5 minutes.
2. Add wine, stir and cook for 1 minute more. Add tomatoes, stir, bring to a boil, cook for 2 minutes, add parsley, stir again and take off heat.

3. Pour this mix into a heat proof dish that fits your air fryer, add fish, season it with salt and pepper and cook in your fryer at 350 degrees F for 14 minutes.
4. Divide fish and tomatoes mix on plates and serve. Enjoy!

Nutrition: calories 231, fat 8, fiber 12, carbs 26, protein 14

Special Catfish Fillets

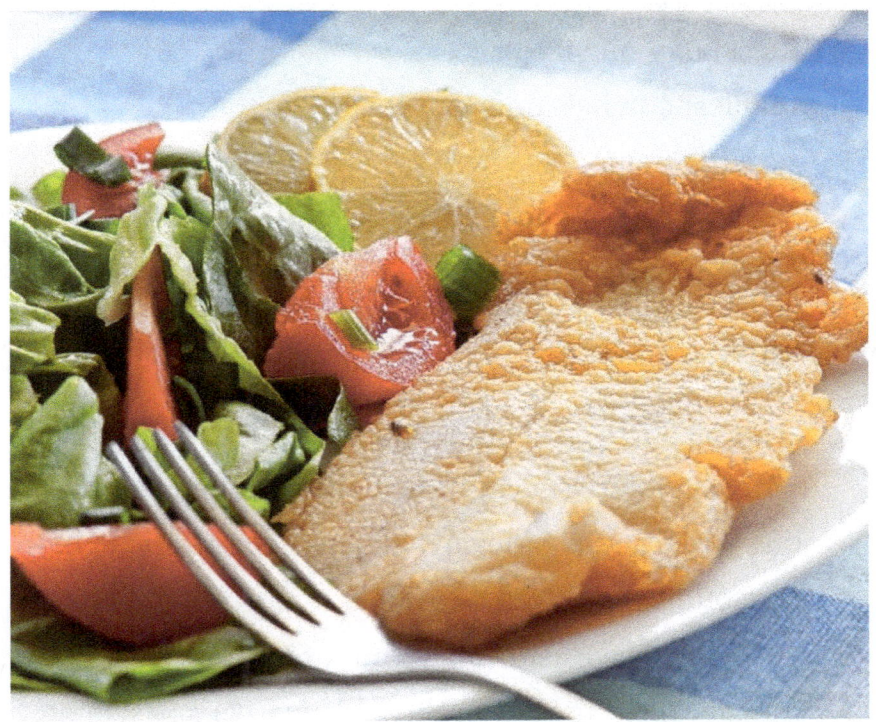

Preparation time: 10 minutes

Cooking time: 12 minutes

Servings: 4

Ingredients:

- 2 catfish fillets
- 1⁄2 teaspoon garlic, minced

- 2 ounces butter
- 4 ounces Worcestershire sauce ½ teaspoon jerk seasoning
- 1 teaspoon mustard
- 1 tablespoon balsamic vinegar
- ¾ cup catsup
- Salt and black pepper to the taste 1 tablespoon parsley, chopped

Directions:

1. Heat up a pan with the butter over medium heat, add Worcestershire sauce, garlic, jerk seasoning, mustard, catsup, vinegar, salt and pepper, stir well, take off heat and add fish fillets.
2. Toss well, leave aside for 10 minutes, drain fillets, transfer them to your preheated air fryer's basket at 350 degrees F and cook for 8 minutes, flipping fillets halfway.
3. Divide among plates, sprinkle parsley on top and serve right away. Enjoy!

Nutrition: calories 351, fat 8, fiber 16, carbs 27, protein 17

Coconut Tilapia

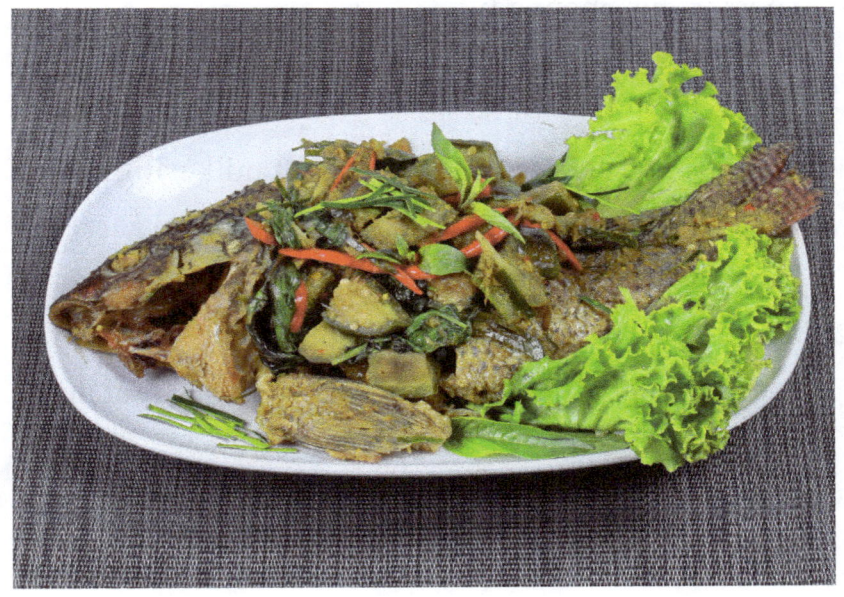

Preparation time: 10 minutes

Cooking time: 10 minutes

Servings: 4

Ingredients:

- 4 medium tilapia fillets
- Salt and black pepper to the taste ½ cup coconut milk
- 1 teaspoon ginger, grated

- ½ cup cilantro, chopped
- 2 garlic cloves, chopped
- ½ teaspoon garam masala Cooking spray
- ½ jalapeno, chopped

Directions:

1. In your food processor, mix coconut milk with salt, pepper, cilantro, ginger, garlic, jalapeno and garam masala and pulse really well.
2. Spray fish with cooking spray, spread coconut mix all over, rub well, transfer to your air fryer's basket and cook at 400 degrees F for 10 minutes.
3. Divide among plates and serve hot.
    Enjoy!

Nutrition: calories 200, fat 5, fiber 6, carbs 25, protein 26

Tilapia and Chives Sauce

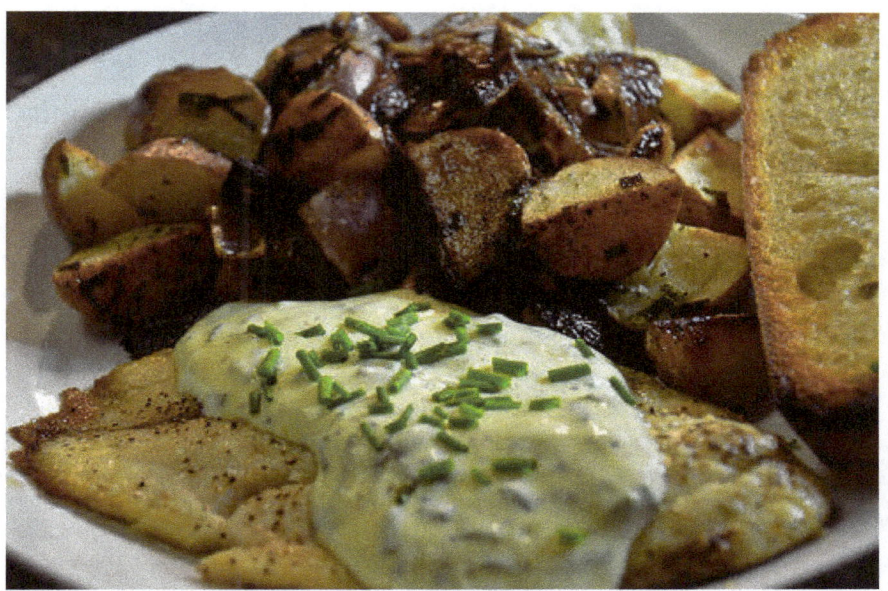

Preparation time: 10 minutes

Cooking time: 8 minutes

Servings: 4

Ingredients:

- 4 medium tilapia fillets
- Cooking spray
- Salt and black pepper to the taste 2 teaspoons honey
- ¼ cup Greek yogur
- Juice from 1 lemon

- 2 tablespoons chives, chopped

Directions:

1. Season fish with salt and pepper, spray with cooking spray, place in preheated air fryer 350 degrees F and cook for 8 minutes, flipping halfway.
2. Meanwhile, in a bowl, mix yogurt with honey, salt, pepper, chives and lemon juice and whisk really well.
3. Divide air fryer fish on plates, drizzle yogurt sauce all over and serve right away.
   Enjoy!

Nutrition: calories 261, fat 8, fiber 18, carbs 24, protein 21

Honey Sea Bass

Preparation time: 10 minutes

Cooking time: 10 minutes

Servings: 2

Ingredients:

- 2 sea bass fillets
- Zest from 1/2 orange, grated
- Juice from 1/2 orange
- A pinch of salt and black pepper
- 2 tablespoons mustard
- 2 teaspoons honey
- 2 tablespoons olive oil
- 1/2 pound canned lentils, drained
- A small bunch of dill, chopped
- 2 ounces watercress
- A small bunch of parsley, chopped

Directions:

1. Season fish fillets with salt and pepper, add orange zest and juice, rub with 1 tablespoon oil, with honey and mustard, rub, transfer to your air fryer and cook at 350 degrees F for 10 minutes, flipping halfway.

2. Meanwhile, put lentils in a small pot, warm it up over medium heat, add the rest of the oil, watercress, dill and parsley, stir well and divide among plates.
3. Add fish fillets and serve right away. Enjoy!

Nutrition: calories 212, fat 8, fiber 12, carbs 9, protein 17

Tasty Pollock

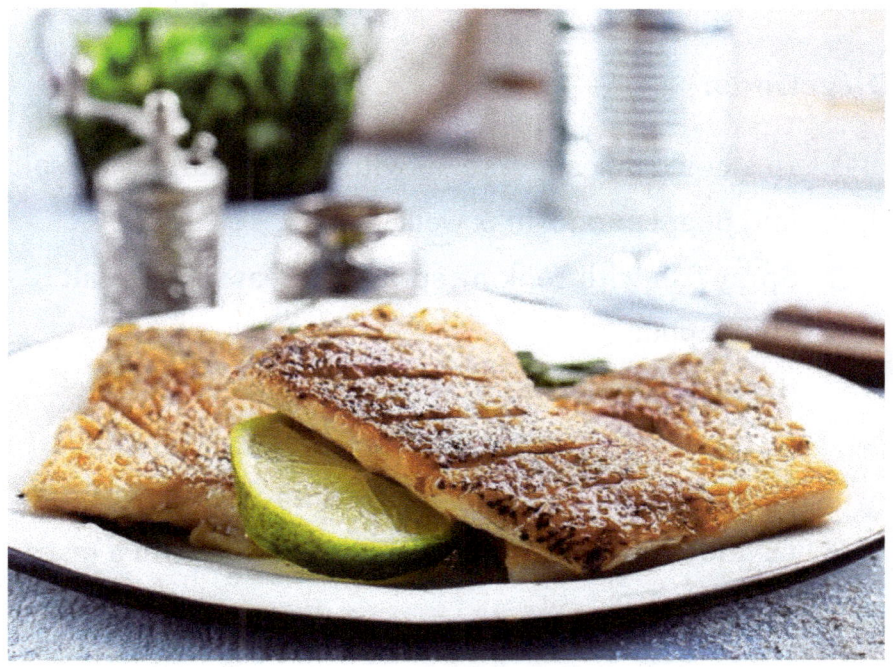

Preparation time: 10 minutes

Cooking time: 15 minutes

Servings: 6

Ingredients:

- ½ cup sour cream
- 4 Pollock fillets, boneless
- ¼ cup parmesan, grated

- 2 tablespoons butter, melted
- Salt and black pepper to the taste Cooking spray

Directions:

1. In a bowl, mix sour cream with butter, parmesan, salt and pepper and whisk well.
2. Spray fish with cooking spray and season with salt and pepper.
   Spread sour cream mix on one side of each Pollock fillet, arrange them in your preheated air fryer at 320 degrees F and cook them for 15 minutes.
3. Divide Pollock fillets on plates and serve with a tasty side salad. Enjoy!

Nutrition: calories 300, fat 13, fiber 3, carbs 14, protein 44

Buttered Shrimp Skewers

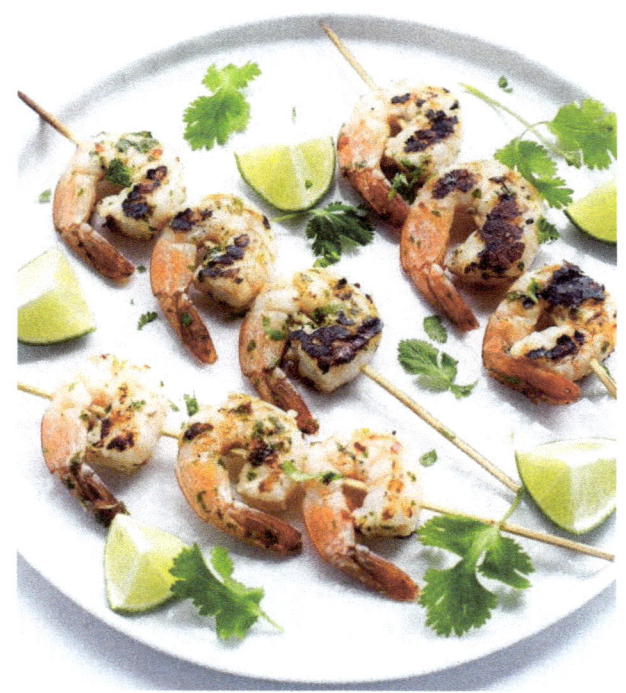

Preparation time: 10 minutes

Cooking time: 6 minutes

Servings: 2

Ingredients:

- 8 shrimps, peeled and deveined 4 garlic cloves, minced

- Salt and black pepper to the taste 8 green bell pepper slices
- 1 tablespoon rosemary, chopped 1 tablespoon butter, melted

Directions:

√ In a bowl, mix shrimp with garlic, butter, salt, pepper, rosemary and bell pepper slices, toss to coat and leave aside for 10 minutes.

√ Arrange 2 shrimp and 2 bell pepper slices on a skewer and repeat with the rest of the shrimp and bell pepper pieces.

√ Place them all in your air fryer's basket and cook at 360 degrees F for 6 minutes.

√ Divide among plates and serve right away.

Enjoy!

Nutrition: calories 140, fat 1, fiber 12, carbs 15, protein 7

Asian Salmon

Preparation time: 1 hour

Cooking time: 15 minutes

Servings: 2

Ingredients:

- 2 medium salmon fillets
- 6 tablespoons light soy sauce 3 teaspoons mirin
- 1 teaspoon water
- 6 tablespoons honey

Directions:

√ In a bowl, mix soy sauce with honey, water and mirin, whisk well, add salmon, rub well and leave aside in the fridge for 1 hour.

√ Transfer salmon to your air fryer and cook at 360 degrees F for 15 minutes, flipping them after 7 minutes.

√ Meanwhile, put the soy marinade in a pan, heat up over medium heat, whisk well, cook for 2 minutes and take off heat.

√ Divide salmon on plates, drizzle marinade all over and serve.

Enjoy!

Nutrition: calories 300, fat 12, fiber 8, carbs 13, protein 24

Cod Steaks with Plum Sauce

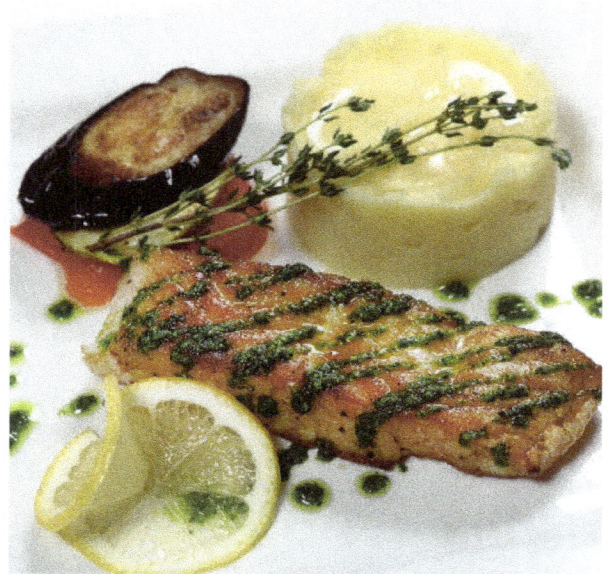

Preparation time: 10 minutes

Cooking time: 20 minutes

Servings: 2

Ingredients:

- 2 big cod steaks
- Salt and black pepper to the taste 1/2 teaspoon garlic powder
- 1/2 teaspoon ginger powder
- 1/4 teaspoon turmeric powder

- 1 tablespoon plum sauce Cooking spray

Directions:

√ Season cod steaks with salt and pepper, spray them with cooking oil, add garlic powder, ginger powder and turmeric powder and rub well.
√ Place cod steaks in your air fryer and cook at 360 degrees F for 15 minutes, flipping them after 7 minutes.
√ Heat up a pan over medium heat, add plum sauce, stir and cook for 2 minutes. Divide cod steaks on plates, drizzle plum sauce all over and serve.

Enjoy!

Nutrition: calories 250, fat 7, fiber 1, carbs 14, protein 12

Flavored Air Fried Salmon

Preparation time: 1 hour

Cooking time: 8 minutes

Servings: 2

Ingredients:

- 2 salmon fillets
- 2 tablespoons lemon juice
- Salt and black pepper to the taste 1/2 teaspoon garlic powder
- 1/3 cup water
- 1/3 cup soy sauce
- 3 scallions, chopped
- 1/3 cup brown sugar
- 2 tablespoons olive oil

Directions:

√ In a bowl, mix sugar with water, soy sauce, garlic powder, salt, pepper, oil and lemon juice, whisk well, add salmon fillets, toss to coat and leave aside in the fridge for 1 hour.
√ Transfer salmon fillets to the fryer's basket and cook at 360 degrees F for 8 minutes flipping them halfway.

√ Divide salmon on plates, sprinkle scallions on top and serve right away.

Enjoy!

Nutrition: calories 300, fat 12, fiber 10, carbs 23, protein 20

Salmon with Capers and Mash

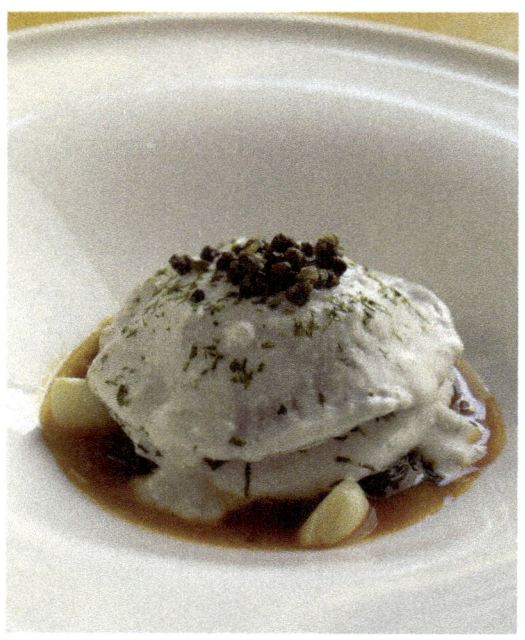

Preparation time: 10 minutes

Cooking time: 20 minutes

Servings: 4

Ingredients:

- 4 salmon fillets, skinless and boneless 1 tablespoon capers, drained
  Salt and black pepper to the taste Juice from 1 lemon
- 2 teaspoons olive oil

- *For the potato mash:*
- 2 tablespoons olive oil

  1 tablespoon dill, dried

  1 pound potatoes, chopped 1/2 cup milk

Directions:

- Put potatoes in a pot, add water to cover, add some salt, bring to a boil over medium high heat, cook for 15 minutes, drain, transfer to a bowl, mash with a potato masher, add 2 tablespoons oil, dill, salt, pepper and milk, whisk well and leave aside for now.
- Season salmon with salt and pepper, drizzle 2 teaspoons oil over them, rub, transfer to your air fryer's basket, add capers on top, cook at 360 degrees F and cook for 8 minutes.

  Divide salmon and capers on plates, add mashed potatoes on the side, drizzle lemon juice all over and serve.

Enjoy!

Nutrition: calories 300, fat 17, fiber 8, carbs 12, protein 18

CPSIA information can be obtained
at www.ICGtesting.com
Printed in the USA
LVHW082056270621
691285LV00007B/283